Overeating? : Stop Overeating, Binge Eating, & Get The Natural Slim Body You Deserve

A self-help guide to control emotional eating today!

Samantha Michaels

Table of Contents

Chapter 1: Understanding Binge Eating Disorder

Have you ever felt a strange craving for food you haven't eaten in a while? Sometimes, you might decide to indulge your craving, and find yourself overeating too quickly until you're too full you feel like your stomach is going to burst. Congratulations, you've just experienced binge eating.

Occasional overeating does not pose much of a problem, but it can soon lead to habitual binge eating that can already be considered a form of eating disorder.

What Is Binge Eating Disorder (BED)?

The term "binge" means excessive indulgence, and was used originally to refer to excessive drinking. Today, we use it more often to refer to binge eating, or compulsive eating which leads to consuming too much food in a short time.

Binge eating is considered one of the most common eating disorders at present. If unchecked, it becomes a serious health problem as it eventually leads to obesity and other ailments like diabetes, heart diseases, gastrointestinal problems, and even certain types of cancer.

Symptoms of a Binge

A person who has developed a serious case of binge eating disorder may experience one or more of the following symptoms:

- Frequent binge eating episodes, characterized by trancelike rapid food intake until your stomach feels uncomfortable.
- Stress and agitation that can only be cured by food.
- Inability to control what you eat and how much.
- Compulsive overeating even when you don't really feel hungry, sometimes even throughout the entire day.

- Eating a lot of food in secret, because you don't want to be seen consuming all that food in your plate.
- You feel guilty, depressed, or disgusted with yourself afterward.

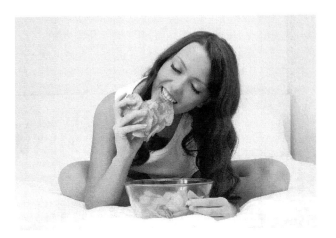

How You Feel During a Binge

Moments before you experience a binge, you might feel a craving so intense for a certain food. Minutes stretch into hours as you attempt to get to the food stash, and you feel more agitated with each moment. You've got to eat, and you've got to eat now!

Then, when the food is in front of you, it begins. You might not notice the amount of food you are consuming, because you are too focused on savoring what you eat: the taste, the textures, and you lose yourself in that sensation.

You just feel the need to eat, and eat, and eat, forgetting table manners and stuffing the food in your mouth almost mechanically, as if you are going to die if you can't have that next bite. It's like your stomach has turned to a bottomless pit that you can't fill.

You don't notice how quickly the food is disappearing from your plate. It's almost like you're in a trance: you don't know what you're doing and you can't seem to control it. Then, once the episode is over and you've had enough, it hits you. You realize just how much you've eaten, and that's when the negative feelings set in.

What Happens To Your Body When You Binge?

If you have exhibited any of these symptoms and felt exactly that same way described above, there's no need to panic or feel even more guilty or depressed. Remember that there is a cure to every disorder — you just need the mindset to overcome binge eating.

After you have aptly diagnosed your problem, the first step in curing yourself is to go to the root of the problem. You need to understand what causes you to binge.

Scientifically speaking, people who undergo frequent binge eating episodes are unable to break a behavioral and physiological cycle that the body experiences: the binge eating cycle.

First, when you consume a lot of food in a short time, this causes a sudden surge in your body's blood sugar levels. This spike in your blood sugar then sends a message to your pancreas to create more insulin, the hormone that helps break down fat and carbohydrates in food.

However, the sudden release of more insulin causes your blood sugar level to fall. This fall of your blood sugar makes your brain think that you need more food to increase your blood sugar.

So, instead of feeling full, your cravings intensify, particularly for starchy and sugary foods. You keep eating even when you're not physically hungry anymore. As you consume more sugary foods, your blood sugar levels increase again, and the cycle begins again.

This is why binge eating is very difficult to overcome, especially if the severity of the binge episodes has intensified to uncontrollable levels.

Causes of Binge Eating

There are a lot of factors — most of them psychosocial — which might cause a person to develop binge eating disorder. More often than not, people who acquire this condition are people who are experiencing emotional downs, and binge eating becomes a form of coping mechanism for negative experiences in life.

Here are some of the main causes of this disorder:

- Stress. While stress is a normal part of our daily activities, experiencing sudden stressful events such as losing your job or a loved one's death may cause emotional trauma that leads to emotional eating. The same is true if work or school has become too stressful, such as when an exam is approaching or if your boss has given you a lot of work to do.
- Depression. Studies have shown that half of binge eaters have experienced depression sometime during their life. The exact nature of the relationship between depression and eating disorders is unclear — if binge eating is caused by depression or vice versa.
- Low self-esteem. People with low self-esteem often seek refuge in food, and are more likely to develop a form of eating disorder than people with normal self-esteem. Because they feel unaccepted and awkward in social situations, food becomes a form of escape for them.
- Personal problems. In some ways, binge eating is similar to typical addictive behavior to substances like alcohol and drugs. People who can't find a way to solve their problems and who feel helpless tend to escape those problems by overeating.
- Negative emotions. Studies have shown that emotional eating episodes are often triggered by negative emotions, such as anger, loneliness, boredom, or anxiety.
- Behavioral factors. Certain behavioral problems may also trigger binge eating, including impulsiveness, escapist tendencies, irresponsibility and substance abuse.
- Dieting. Although there are no conclusive studies yet that solidly link dieting to binge eating, many people who have undergone excessive dieting claim that it was the deprivation of food which caused them to have emotional eating episodes. Binge eating is also often a result of a failed dieting regimen.

Dieting: The Culprit, Not the Cure

Overweight and obese people are often looking for new dieting fads and regimens to lose weight. However, if the statistics are any indication, excessive dieting often leads to the development of an eating disorder like binge eating.

These are the reasons dieting will never cure obesity and instead cause eating disorders:

- Often than not, a diet and weight loss regimen often entail "cutting down" on your carbohydrates and daily caloric intake. Some diets, like the "after-six" diet even recommend skipping on meals and avoiding certain food types, even those necessary for the body to function well.
- Diets never work because they are often composed of unhealthy weight loss methods focused on excessive exercise and food and nutrient deprivation, which cause you more harm than good.
- Diets are difficult. Most diet regimens are impossible to follow, and not recommended as a permanent lifestyle. They are often short-term fixes which leaves you in a worse state than you were before you started the diet.
- The deprivation caused by dieting heightens your risk to develop binge eating and other eating disorders. It intensifies your hunger and cravings to the point that it triggers compulsive overeating.
- Diets are prone to failure. Because of a diet's rigid menu structure, people who indulge in them tend to get bored or lose interest halfway through the diet plan and revert to their old dieting patterns.
- Dieting doesn't go to the root of your eating and weight problem. It only addresses behavioral problems, and not the psychosocial and emotional aspects which are often the cause of obesity.
- Dieting makes you too obsessed about the physical results: what you see in the mirror and what the weighing scale tells you. Then, when you get the results that you want, you stop doing the regimen, and all that "self-control" is forgotten. Conversely, if you fail to achieve your target, you end up being depressed.

Remember: dieting is never the cure to obesity. If you have been involved in different diets in the past, you know that they never work, and may have in fact contributed to the development of your binge eating disorder.

Who Are Prone To Develop Binge Eating Disorder?
- Women are more likely to develop binge eating disorder than men. At present, 3.5% of American women have developed this disorder, while it affects only 2% of the men.
- 30% of dieters and people who undergo weight management training are said to have binge eating disorder. A person who indulges in dieting is said to be eight times more likely to develop an eating disorder.
- Teenage girls are also more prone to develop this disorder due to excessive dieting.
- Overweight and obese people are also more likely to have this disorder than normal-weight people.

Different Types of Binges

Binge eating disorder and compulsive overeating are only some of several eating disorders that a person can develop. Other eating disorders and behaviors that also involve some type of binges include:
- Night Eating Disorder (NED). People with this disorder tend to skip breakfast and eat little throughout the day. Then, they pack all the calories they need during the night, causing sleep problems and obesity in the long run. Some binge eaters call this the half-binge, which usually takes place at night.
- Bulimia Nervosa. Similar to binge eating, bulimic people tend to have intense cravings for food and stuff themselves full. The difference is that they also have a strong urge to throw up almost immediately after eating.
- Emotional overeating. You only have binge eating episodes when you are upset, depressed or angry. Eating comforts and relaxes you.

- Stress overeating. Binge episodes that are triggered by stress and overwork, often as a way to "unwind" and "relax."
- Sugar addiction. Because the binge eating cycle demands a high amount of glucose on some of its stages, some binge eaters develop intense cravings for sweets.

Binge Eating Is a Behavioral Disorder

Even if you have diagnosed yourself with binge eating disorder, you still might not be able to stop yourself. This is because your body has become accustomed to this behavior, and it's become compulsive for you.

Even when you are conscious of binge eating, you can't break the binge eating cycle that your body undergoes. It has become a habit—a physical and psychological habit that has tripped your body's system and your brain can't seem to do anything about it.

You can't stop binge eating disorder even if you know you have it because you are essentially "addicted" to food. People who develop this disorder tend to release more dopamine (a hormone associated with the reward circuits of the brain, making you "feel good") in response to food intake. This is the same physical reaction that addicts get from alcohol and drug intake.

Conventional Therapy for Binges

Curing eating disorders like binge eating is pretty much a hit-and-miss ordeal. There aren't any extensive studies which will tell you for sure how to stop binge eating. Often, psychiatrists will recommend that you undergo some form of therapy, such as:

- Nutrition counseling – treatment is focused on ingraining the importance of healthy eating and a balanced diet. You will be given advice on your eating habits.
- Cognitive-behavioral therapy – treatment that intends to change your habits and mindset about food and eating, to transform negative behavior patterns into positive and healthy ones.
- Dialectical behavior therapy – this is similar to cognitive-behavioral therapy, but it is more focused on improving

your self-image, accepting yourself and how to handle stress and negative emotions positively.

You may be given a combination of group and individual therapy sessions on all these types of therapy for binge eating. Sometimes, families and friends are also included in a session if social factors have been determined as a cause of the disorder. If nothing works, however, you will be given several medicines to help manage the disorder, including antidepressants and anti-anxiety drugs.

However, many patients report that therapies often fail them — especially for obese patients. Research even suggests that these forms of therapy fail dismally in eliminating binge eating problems in an individual, although they seem to work initially.

It's unclear why therapies fail to address binge eating problems, but experts have a guess:

Say, after a few sessions, you feel better and in control of your eating urges and cravings. You stop the therapy entirely. However, once therapy is over, you are confronted everyday with your greatest weakness: food. Unlike alcoholics and drug dependents that can stay away from their addictive substance, you, binge eater, must face your devils every day to survive.

This is when relapse commonly occurs. After a month or so, you will soon find yourself slipping back to the old habits.

Chapter 2: Introduction to Hunger-Directed Eating

While prospects for curing and overcoming binge eating seem hopeless, there's no reason to feel depressed about it. In recent years, there have been different ways that binge eaters have discovered to conquer this disorder.

Since therapy and other short-term fixes don't seem to do the trick, the solution to stop binge eating is obvious: you need a lifestyle change, particularly in your eating habits. You need to make changes, but these changes must not be temporary; you need to be committed to make these changes permanent.

The switch will be gradual, step-by-step. Sudden changes won't benefit you at the least. But what will you change? There are so many diet shifts to choose from. One of the most recommended ways to beat binge eating is to re-learn instinctive eating — in other words, eating only when you are physically hungry.

This eating pattern is also known as hunger-directed eating (HDE). Instead of letting your weighing scale or your cravings dictate what and when you will eat and how much, this technique teaches you to listen to your baser instincts of hunger.

Due to the sensory overload they experience every day, most people forget how being hungry really feels like. This is especially true for binge eaters, who tend to be "food suggestible," or easily lured into eating by the sight and smell of food, even when they are not really hungry. People who have also been engaged in diet and weight loss training also tend to be physically disconnected from feeling hungry.

Wanting to eat and needing to eat are two different things, and this technique will teach you how.

Here's how and why HDE works:
- When you listen to your hunger to direct your eating habits, you become more in control of yourself. You're

sure that you're hungry, and you won't be asking why you need to eat or feel guilty for eating.

- Food tastes better when you are hungry.
- Eating becomes more pleasurable instead of being mechanical, which is the case for binge eaters.
- When you eat when you're hungry, you will more likely crave foods that your body needs instead of junk food and sugary foods.
- You can enjoy sweets occasionally for dessert and not as an entire oversized meal, because you had a filling meal that satisfied your hunger.
- You feel better after a hunger-directed meal rather than feeling unsatisfied, guilty or depressed.
- Listening to your body for signs of hunger is a great way to reach your ideal weight, instead of obsessing over a weighing scale.

How to Listen To Your Hunger

The problem with binge eating is that you have been wired to feel hungry all the time, even when you are not. In contrast, other people seldom feel hungry, or simply fail to identify what hunger feels like.

In order to know if you're hungry or not, you need to look for certain signals from your body. Some experts suggest doing a "mind-body scan," or using your mind to inspect your body for these hunger signs.

First, you need to focus your attention to your body. Avoid doing the scan in front of a food and other stimuli, since these can send your mind mixed signals about how you feel. You need to be calm—take a few deep breaths if needed, and slowly focus on your physical sensations: your stomach, and for other signs such as a weakness of some sort, or a light-headed sensation.

Hunger signs to look for:
- Stomach grumbling
- Hunger pangs, feeling empty or hollow
- Weakness or tiredness

- Difficulty concentrating
- Feeling irritable
- Light-headedness
- Headache
- Shaking

Experts have devised a "hunger scale" to serve as an eating guide for people who are following the HDE (see figure 2.1 above). It's recommended to eat at the first signs of hunger, and to stop eating when you're full (just about two to three handfuls of food, nothing more). Never allow yourself to reach the level 1 in the scale, since eating on a totally empty stomach usually leads to binge eating.

Mind Over Matter: 5 Ways To Trick Your Brain To Stop the Binge

Aside from allowing your hunger to direct your eating habits, here are some quick fixes you can do to avoid binge eating:

1. Eat on a smaller plate. Using a smaller plate tricks your mind into thinking you are eating a lot. Compare it yourself: the same amount of food placed in a big plate and a smaller one. You will see that the amount of food looks more than it really is in a smaller plate.

2. Drink a glass of water before you eat. Water helps cleanse your stomach to prepare it for your next meal, and it also helps create a feeling of fullness on your stomach. Also, have a glass of water beside you while you eat, and alternate every few bites with a few sips of water.

3. Focus on eating. Many people who develop eating disorders are those who are not paying attention to what they're eating. When your mind is elsewhere (such as watching TV), you lose track of how much food you are consuming, and tend to eat more than you normally would have.

    Focus on the food in front of you. Before you eat, take a few deep breaths and relax yourself—that will release some of the tension you are feeling because of hunger. It will also help you avoid going into a trancelike state where you cannot control yourself.

Eat slowly and savor every bite. It takes a while for the brain to register the fullness of your stomach, and slower food intake ensures you don't eat more than you need.

4. Indulge occasionally. Moderation is the key to avoiding binge eating. It is okay to eat the occasional sweet treat or starchy food, but not as a full meal. Eat only a small piece, and only after you have eaten a full, satisfying meal. Consider it a reward for your good work at controlling your hunger.

5. Choose satisfying, healthy foods. Throw out the junk you're keeping in a secret stash. Getting rid of your binge eating disorder means committing yourself fully, and you can't do that with too much temptation at arm's reach.

   When choosing your produce, stay organic where possible. Opt for whole grains instead of processed pasta and other starchy, sugary foods available at the supermarket. Gradually add vegetables to your meals instead of all-meat preparations.

Remember: a balanced diet of healthy carbohydrates, proteins and fats will keep your body running without causing your mind to go haywire.

Chapter 3: How to Stay Thin Eating What You Want

Binge eating disorder and obesity tend to go hand-in-hand, with one disorder leading to the other. Thus, a true solution to these conditions would have to deal with both of them at the same time.

You don't need to starve yourself on unhealthy diet programs which tell you to deprive yourself of your much-needed calories and nutrients. Neither do you have to enroll yourself in a rigorous exercising program which could leave you exhausted and drained of energy.

Forget fad programs — they never work in the long run. Did you know that the popular weight-loss training reality show, "The Biggest Loser," never really worked for the participants? Just a few months after the show, winners of the show tend to regain the weight they lost and even more — further proof that diet regimes involving food deprivation and over-exercising will do you more harm than good.

Unlike what most diet programs will tell you, you don't need to stop eating your favorite foods in order to lose the excess weight. It's never healthy to skip out on important food groups just because they are "fattening."

Thin people will tell you that dieting is never the solution. Here are some of the key secrets to staying thin but still getting to eat what you want:

1. If you're obese, stop obsessing on the scales. The social standards of being thin and being fat border on the ludicrous. Plus, you can't expect to lose all that excess weight at once; excessive and sudden weight loss is never healthy.

   Set a more realistic goal for yourself, but don't obsess if you don't reach it. It's important to be focused on the results you are getting instead of getting depressed because "it's not working well" for you. You'll only relapse to over eating if you do.

2. Have a positive mindset. You can overcome those binges! Maybe not at once, and maybe not after months of hard work on your part, but now that you know what causes it and how you can control it, you are already at an advantage.

3. Don't skip on meals, especially breakfast. Again, quit listening to those fad diet programs. Skipping out on the most important meal of the day won't make you thinner. Breakfast is the meal which gives our body the energy to go through the day, and skipping this meal will only make you hungrier later during lunch or dinner.

4. Moderate what you eat. Instead of stockpiling an entire buffet in your plate, eat smaller portions of a balanced meal. You can do this by gradually decreasing the amount of your food and sticking with that portion. Use a smaller plate and avoid seconds (or thirds). As long as you remain focused on your food, you can avoid craving for more!

5. Eat everything you want. Stop listening to those diet gurus who prescribe what you should and should not eat. Avoiding an "unhealthy" food item is the worst thing you could do to intensify your cravings for it. Instead, if you find yourself craving for cake or ice cream, go get yourself some—but only a small portion, and stop there.
    If you feel yourself craving for more, try to veer your mind away from food and think of something else to do to distract you.

6. Avoid excessive snacking. Even if you're not binge eating anymore, you might still be overeating if you keep snacking between meals, since you're essentially eating more than your body needs to keep it going. If and when you snack, make it as healthy as possible, such as a piece of fruit.

7. Improve your lifestyle. You can't expect to lose weight if you're lazing the whole day away. If you don't have an active lifestyle, you're unlikely to achieve your desired weight. Plan daily activities to keep going, and make sure

you get enough sleep (6-8 hours) to recover from daily stress.

8. Drink water. 6-8 glasses of water per day can do wonders for your health.

9. Enjoy your food. When you take time to savor the food you eat, the less likely you will binge. Conversely, you can't enjoy eating if you're depriving yourself of certain foods. Learn to strike a balance on the kinds of food you eat, and stop depriving yourself unnecessarily.

Psychology of eating: why satisfaction and moderation will get you better results than deprivation

Eating disorders like over eating and emotional eating are a direct result of different factors which cause an individual to have a skewed idea about him or herself. It is a psychological problem that can lead to further complications that may endanger a person's life.

People with eating disorders never benefit from diet regimes. In fact, eating disorders often stem with a person's need to be accepted by society through rigorous dieting. It's a fact: the prevalent culture of deprivation and stinginess that society connects with the ideal concept of beauty and attractiveness is causing misery to thousands of men and women at present.

Curing binge eating disorder entails going against this social norm. You should indulge and satisfy your needs instead of depriving them. As long as you maintain a moderate intake of foods that satisfy you, you will soon be able to overcome these binges.

Chapter 4: Ending Your Meals with Ease

Stopping binge eating is a great challenge, but you will definitely feel better once you have resumed eating normally. Eating a full meal—nothing more, nothing less—will make you feel satisfied and happy, unlike binge episodes where you never seem to get enough and leave you feeling frustrated or guilty afterward.

Another key to ending your over eating and emotional eating episodes is to know when to stop eating. Earlier in this book, we have discussed hunger-directed eating and how you can detect physical signs of hunger. This time, we will be discussing how you can detect signs of fullness and how to know you have eaten enough to fuel your activities until your next meal.

Signs of Fullness

Being mindful of what you eat is a crucial step in stopping binge eating. That's why eating needs your entire attention. Stop eating in front of the TV! Put down that book that you're reading!

You see, the sensation of fullness doesn't come from the actual fullness of your stomach. Instead, it's the result of a chemical reaction in your brain after you have put something in your stomach. This feeling lasts for 3-5 hours — just enough until your next meal.

Binges are unsatisfying because instead of this chemical reaction, your brain is releasing the feel-good hormone dopamine during a binge episode. Dopamine makes you crave more instead of making you feel satiated.

Here are some tips on how to look for signs that you have eaten enough:

- Time your meal. The average time it takes for the brain to register feelings of fullness is 20 minutes. After 20 minutes, try doing the mind-body scan again and see if the hunger has dissipated. You might still want to eat more at this point, but before you do, check for other signs of fullness.

- Put your fork down after a few bites or so. It can take a while before you begin to feel the sensation of fullness, and eating slowly will help you to notice it more quickly than if you were gorging on food.
- A sign of fullness is when you no longer feel any physical symptom indicating hunger, and when you have a general feeling of contentment. If you stopped eating and end up obsessing whether you're full or not, that's probably an indication that you're not really full yet.
- Your mind begins to wander when you're full, and what you're eating doesn't seem to taste as good as at the beginning of your meal.
- You don't feel bloated. The sensation of being bloated is an indication that you may have eaten too much again. Comfortable fullness doesn't make you feel weighed down.

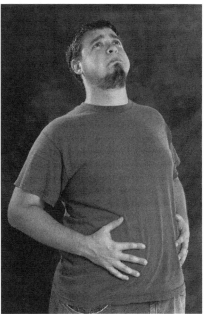

Comfortable fullness, not feeling bloated

End a Meal with Ease after Your Hunger Is Appeased

Once your hunger is dissipated and the feeling of fullness sets in, you should be prepared to stop eating. Binge eaters will most likely struggle at this point, as your body has been accustomed to having binge episodes. It will take time and practice to have a perfectly balanced, moderately-proportioned meal.

Don't give in to the craving to eat more—you will endanger yourself from having yet another binge episode. Instead, try one of the following tips to end your craving for more food:

- Have dessert. Eating something sweet can help give you a slight sugar rush enough to stabilize your blood sugar levels and break the binge eating cycle. It also helps control your cravings. While you can have some cake or cookie occasionally, train yourself to choose something healthier, such as berries, watermelon, or other fruits that have high water content.
- Peppermint works wonders. The herb peppermint is a natural appetite suppressant which could help you manage your eating habits, and control your cravings for more servings. It can be a piece of gum or candy, and even a hot cup of tea. Peppermint-flavored mouthwash will also work.
- Move away from the sight of food. It's best to avoid temptation at this point, so it's probably better if you went to the bedroom or the living room and distract yourself with a good movie. Or, you can take a nice, leisurely walk around the neighborhood — it will be a good distraction and the movement will help you digest your meal better.
- Plan your activities. If the urge to have seconds is so strong, you will need to have something to distract you immediately after the meal. Even a simple act as cleaning your room or checking your mail can help you keep away from food.

Chapter 5: Will Power and Want Power

Now that you know some basic tricks to help you control your cravings and how much you eat for each meal, the next step would be to understand what you need to successfully overcome your binge episodes: Will power.

You might think that will power is just a metaphysical concept that people use in order to motivate you into doing something. On the contrary, will power has a scientific basis, and can actually be developed and improved.

Developing your will power is necessary if you truly wish to defeat those cravings and stop your over eating habits. There will be lots of times when you just want to give up and give in to your cravings, and there will be a lot of times when you will lose the battle. Don't worry; that's all part of the learning process of strengthening your will power.

Will power is that physical and mental trick you can pull when the urge to have a second serving hits. It helps you to say "no" even when your body is screaming "yes, yes, I want that next piece!"

So where does will power come from? The prefrontal cortex (PFT) (see fig. 5.1 below) of our brain is said to be the core of this ability of humans to do something that they normally do not want to do.

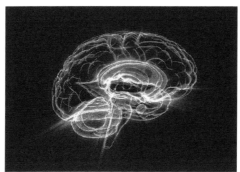

The prefrontal cortex, responsible for a person's will power.

The PFT is often likened to a "policeman" in a person's brain, because it aids in the process of selecting the best options and decisions in any given situation. It analyzes any known and related data in order to predict outcomes of certain situations.

To illustrate, consider this situation: should you binge eat or control your cravings? Even if your body has become hooked to the binge eating cycle, the PFT is the part of your brain which knows and understands that binge eating cannot be healthy for you, and it will order you to stop. That's why binge eaters are often conflicted — they know what they "should" do, but their body fails to obey the PFT's order.

Why does this happen? Why most of the time, will power loses to a stronger desire, the "want" power? This is because will power isn't innate and constant — its strength varies depending on several conditions:

Why Will Power Fails
1. Stress. Yes: will power depletes the more you are confronted with stressful situations, until you finally give in to the inevitable and have that next serving.
2. Lack of nutrition. That's why you were never able to follow your diet program, and why it never worked for you. Since your body hasn't been getting the right nutrition for a long time, it has contributed to your lack of will power to follow through with your diet plan.
3. Lack of sleep. Sleep deprivation affects your entire brain, including the PFT. That's probably the reason why you can't seem to make sound choices after you've been awake for extended hours of the day.
4. Lack of energy. When your energy level goes down, so does your will power. Research even suggests that will power is strongest at the earlier part of the day and depletes as the day ends. This is because you are confronted by decision-making choices throughout the day which use up your will power.

Looking at that list, it's no wonder that you are having difficulties on calling on your will power to stop the binge. Your struggle with binge eating has already robbed you of the essential tools you need to sharpen your will power! It's also why dieting has always failed you, because following a diet plan involves exercising your will power as well.

Thankfully, the strength of a person's will power can be trained, and it can be useful to some extent to stop binge eating episodes entirely.

Training Your Will Power

Studies have shown that a person's will power "reserve" increases with two primary types of activities: exercise and meditation. Here are some things you could do to increase your will power:

1. Meditation exercises. Even just 5 minutes of meditating each day can strengthen your will power over time. Just close your eyes, settle in a relaxed position, and focus your mind on your breathing. Allow your mind to wander. Exercises like yoga will be helpful as well.
2. Muscular tension and reflex control. Studies have proven that people who tighten their muscles when faced with a difficult decision often make the right choices. These include tightening your hands to a fist, gripping something tightly in your hand, or even raising your toes can help you make healthier choices in your eating habits.
3. Keep a journal. A research suggests that people who keep track of their daily choices are able to control themselves more than others who don't.
4. Avoid alcohol. Alcohol lowers your blood glucose levels and sends a message to your brain that you need to eat more. It also lowers your self-awareness and control, making you more prone to a binge episode.
5. Nutritional supplements. Calcium and vitamin D supplements are said to help you control your cravings for fatty foods. Omega3 is also a healthy enzyme you need — deficiency on this enzyme can result to constant hunger.

How to Crave What Is Good For You

In order to control your cravings completely instead of the other way around, you need to understand why you crave certain foods. There are a lot of explanations why we crave, but often than not, cravings are our body's way of saying that we need a certain enzyme or substance that can be found on the food that we're craving. For example, if you crave for ice cream or other dairy foods, you might be running low in calcium.

On the other hand, you might be experiencing an emotional craving, or craving that is triggered by your emotions. This is the common downfall of many binge eaters—and most likely, you will crave for junk food that will only intensify your cravings. Processed carbohydrates, like pasta and pizza, and sugary foods like candies and cookies, are often the subject of such cravings.

How can you overcome these cravings and instead crave for healthier options? Again, it will depend on your will power, but you can make it easier for you to make the better choice using the following tips:

1. Avoid temptation. If you know the unhealthy foods that you crave the most, then it's time to throw it out of your pantry. Remove all junk food from your house—or at least place them in an area out of your reach, such as the attic or the basement, so it'd be difficult to get to them.

2. Substitute. Learning to control your cravings means you should train yourself to be satisfied with healthier options. For instance, if you are craving for sweets, choose fruits instead of candies; if you're craving ice cream, choose yogurt instead, and pickles instead of chips. You'd make it a lot easier if you stock these substitutes instead of the junk you usually crave.

3. Give it an hour. When an intense craving for junk hits you, master yourself and wait for one hour before giving in. Meanwhile, distract yourself from the craving by doing something else. Experts explain that cravings usually last only 20 to 30 minutes, so it will most likely have passed after the hour is up.

4. Treat yourself. If you really need a junk food fix, keep a small emergency stash instead of your usual bulk buys, and have a tiny bite when the craving hits. A scoop of ice

cream instead of a gallon, one chocolate chip cookie instead of an entire box.

5. Brush your teeth. Brushing and washing your mouth helps you quell a craving because it removes previous flavors in your mouth and controls your appetite for more.

Chapter 6: Measuring Your Slim Success with Your Sanity, Not Your Scale

After knowing and understanding the necessary tools you need to stop the overeating e and emotional eating, it's time to get down to the actual struggle. Losing weight is a great goal to set, so long as you don't get too obsessed with what results you want to achieve.

As we've discussed before, most diet plans today are too ideal and impossible to follow. That's why most dieters are doomed to failure even before they've begun a diet regimen. Unless you don't have regular work or school, you can't expect to keep a killer-pace exercise routine or that you won't be exposed to any junk food at all!

Let's face reality, and reality isn't about society's ideal of what is the "normal" weight and shape of a person of your age. Most diet plans are often recommended by celebrities who have personal trainers and exclusive gym club memberships!

In the real world, you can't expect to lose 20 lbs. in one week. You can't change from size 14 to size 6 in just a few days, even if you starve yourself. So, stop obsessing with the weighing scales and get real.

The success of losing weight varies per individual. The same plan won't get the same results for two different people: genetic factors and environmental factors are the reasons why you won't get the same results as someone else will.

It's time to let common sense rule your goal instead of the weighing scale. Common sense will tell you that you can't lose all those pounds overnight. Common sense will tell you that depriving yourself of certain foods will actually be detrimental for your nutritional needs.

And, common sense will tell you that you need to find a better plan to control your cravings and your binges rather than following those sensationalized, bandwagon diet plans.

Here are some tips on creating a realistic lifestyle and nutritional plan that could help you to lose weight:

1. Instead of setting your ideal weight as your goal, focus instead on making behavioral and habitual changes in your food and nutritional plate.

2. Set short-term goals and long-term goals. It's easier to follow a plan when you have short-term goals to look forward to, while not losing sight of your long-term goal. In this case, the long-term goal would be a lifestyle change for your eating habits, through the help of short-term, one-step-at-a-time goals you can achieve in the course of time.

3. Forget skipping out meals and deprivation. If a previous diet has made you fear all those carbs and fats, it's time to change your mindset. These enzymes aren't necessarily bad; in fact, they are essential for your body to function correctly. The proper attitude would be to include these moderately in your daily food plate.

4. Healthy isn't boring. Just because you're eating healthier foods doesn't mean they don't taste as good. You can find great-tasting recipe alternatives online for a healthier version of your favorite dishes.

5. Stay active. You can't become fitter if you're always lying on the couch, watching TV. Along with meal plans, you should also include exercise and other activities which would help you tone your body, as well as other healthy lifestyle changes including getting enough sleep and de-stressing.

6. Do it gradually. That's why you have long-term and short-term goals: because you can't achieve everything overnight. Don't be impatient, and instead mark your progress every week and congratulate yourself for every milestone you've achieved. Start out with small goals that will help you achieve bigger goals.

7. Treat yourself. A reward system is a great motivation to stick with your plan. Along with goals, plan rewards you

can give to yourself after each successful week. It may be a piece of sweet, or any food you crave the most.

Gauge Your Success without the Scale

Remember, humans normally gain and lose weight almost every day due to a number of factors, and it's never a reliable measure for a successful diet and nutritional plan.

Instead of constantly weighing yourself on the scale, try these tips to measure how you are doing with your nutritional plan:

1. Your body tone. You may not be losing weight because your body mass remains the same, but the composition of your body is changing. Look at the mirror. Do your arms look less flabby? You might be losing body fat as they become transformed into healthy muscle.
2. Check your wardrobe. Is it your imagination or are those pants feeling a little bit loose? It means your body is becoming healthier.
3. Stamina and endurance. Are you feeling less out of breath after a 30-minute hike? It means your exercise has been paying off, and your body is functioning better from your healthier food plate and the active lifestyle.

Chapter 7: Self Help Step by Step Plan

So you want to start a plan to end those binges, but you don't know where and when you should begin. This section will guide you with every step of the way until you've managed to control your cravings and stop binge eating entirely.

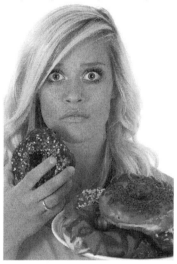

Getting Ready

This is where it all begins. Wanting to quit binge eating and being ready to quit are two different things. You might want to, but your body will probably tell you a different story.

Here is where strengthening your will power will come in. In order to master your urges to over eat, you will need to equip yourself with the necessary skills, and will power is crucial to this.

Start with simple meditation exercises and muscle reflex exercises. This will help you better control yourself, and will help you take that next step forward: committing yourself to make the necessary changes.

This is also when you should create a plan on how you could quit. Refer to the previous section for the guide on what should be included in your plan. Set a reasonable timeframe — maybe 6 months, a year at the most. If you're currently working on a diet or weight loss plan, it's time to drop out—that's not the plan you need right now.

Starting Well

When you've made your plan, the next step is implementation. This is where the real test begins. Planning isn't quite the same as actually quitting.

That's why you need realistic, short-term goals at the beginning of your plan. It may be a simple exercise, such as trying to be conscious during a binge episode instead of being in a trance. Gradually, the goals will change to bigger ones, but for now, focus on reaching those small goals you've set out for yourself.

If you fail to make your first goals, don't be disheartened. Consider it a learning process and make a note of why you failed to reach a goal. Maybe the goal wasn't realistic and you have to make adjustments, or you need to work harder.

Regular Eating

Don't be afraid of food. It might be the kryptonite that makes you go weak and crazy, but it's time to face your fear rather than let it master you. Remember, it's just food—you shouldn't let it rule your life.

Try to establish a good meal plan that you could work with your regular schedule, and stick with it. Keeping food journals at this point will help you keep track of your progress and may motivate you to stick with your goals.

When the cravings hit you, try one of the tricks mentioned earlier to control it. When you do this successfully, you can reward yourself with a little treat.

Alternatives to Binge Eating

Know what triggers you to binge eat, and confront these causes head-on. Solving binge eating doesn't only revolve around your eating behaviors and habits; it often has something to do with your personal disposition as well.

If you're an emotional binge eater, you can choose other activities to relieve yourself instead of resorting to food. Meditation exercises, writing a diary and even calling a friend when you're down can help you control the urge to binge eat.

If stress is your trigger, find other ways to calm yourself. De-stressing exercises like yoga, a soothing cup of tea are great substitutes to donuts and ice cream. Also, take better care of yourself — stress and negative emotions result from unhealthy lifestyle and habits.

Problem Solving

Binge eating isn't the solution to your problems. It's time for you to stop escaping your woes and face them instead. Not only is this escapist tendency unhealthy, in your case it has become destructive.

Instead of obsessing about food, think of the roots of your cravings. Were you feeling especially low or depressed? Did you feel deprived of something you wanted so badly?

Stopping binge eating involves solving the problems that actually causes you to binge. Often, it has little to do with food and everything to do with who you are: self-image, beliefs, social life, and your needs.

These are the things you need to address, and if you need to make changes to solve your issues, don't be afraid to do so.

Body Image

In the end, overcoming binge eating is about respecting and loving who you are. It's about accepting who you are, and by changing the things you don't like about yourself.

Improving your self-image or body image can help a lot to stop those binge episodes. Stop comparing yourself with other people, or thinking about the social standards of beauty and attractiveness.

Remember these affirmations and tell them to yourself when the urge hits you:
- I am my own person.
- I am a beautiful person and I won't let anybody tell me differently.
- Binge eating is not the solution to my problems.
- I am a strong person. I can solve my problems and I will not escape them through eating.

Ending Well

All's well that ends well. Breaking the habit caused by binged eating is difficult, and if you don't do it right, you are in danger of relapsing into your binge episodes again.

The key to ending binge eating forever is to commit to make lifestyle changes, and changing negative behaviors and beliefs into a positive attitude about life. After you've done that, reward yourself a little about your achievements.

Your struggle with food addiction should not remain hovering in your life like a ghost of the past. When you've overcome your binge eating, you should move on and simply learn from your experience with this disorder. After that, you'll never take yourself for granted ever again.

Chapter 8: The Top 70 Ways to Calm Yourself without Food

Binge eating disorder develops when you let food become your escape from all the problems you need to confront every day. It's easier to fall into a habit than to break it, but never believe that you don't have other options.

When you feel that you're getting stressed, angry, or depressed, find other ways to relax and get calm. When the craving for food becomes too strong, here are the top 70 things you could do to distract yourself.

20 Meditation Techniques

Meditation is an excellent way to calm yourself—you just need to learn how to do it properly. Here are the top tips for meditation beginners:

1. Include meditation time on your schedule. Making it a formal activity will allow you to improve over time.
2. Choose where you meditate. Remove yourself from stressful surroundings, and choose a quiet, relaxing room for your meditation.
3. Make sure you won't be disturbed while you meditate.
4. Be comfortable. Settle on a cushion and sit in a relaxed position.
5. Practice deep, slow breathing. It's the basic step needed to meditate, since it relaxes you and focuses your thoughts.
6. Do stretching exercises. It helps release tension from your muscles and allows you to relax easier.
7. Focus on a purpose. Meditation is not passive; it requires active thought and hard work. You should always have a goal in mind before you meditate.
8. Use visual cues. If you have difficulty meditating with your eyes closed, focus your eyes on an object instead.
9. Don't be frustrated or stressed. Emotions like frustration break your line of thought and could make it hard for you to concentrate.

10. Do the mind-body scan. This technique mentioned earlier, which uses the mind to feel parts of your body, is a great way to meditate.

11. Do it long-term. Don't treat meditation as a Band-Aid solution. Instead, consider it a great addition to your lifestyle that helps you relieve stress.

12. Mornings are best for meditation. It's the time when your mind is still clear and free from the stress of daily activities.

13. Appreciate your progress. It will take practice to meditate properly. Congratulate yourself on whatever you achieve with every session.

14. Do it before you eat. Eating makes you feel sleepy, and you might fall asleep if you meditate after eating.

15. Smile. This expression relaxes your facial muscles and lightens your disposition.

16. Do it slowly. Don't rush through meditation mechanically. Enjoy every moment, and let it relax you.

17. Try yoga. It's an excellent exercise to help you meditate better.

18. Try it with music and sounds. Instrumental music or sounds of nature can help you to relax.

19. Read up. Browse meditation books and online resources to help you improve your technique.

20. Get instruction manuals or audiobooks. These materials can guide you throughout your meditation.

20 Ways of Changing Your Thoughts

Positive thinking and attitude will help you achieve your goals. Here are 20 sure tips to change your thoughts positively.

1. Find humor in everything. This can help you see things differently for once and stops the onslaught of negative emotions that result to over eating and emotional eating.

2. Stop putting yourself down. Having a negative inner voice can make you pretty depressed even without reason.

3. Use positive words. These are words that make you happy instead of words that make you sad or angry.

4. Analyze. When things go wrong, stop taking the blame. Instead, think on all the factors and why those things happened.

5. Accept your mistakes. You aren't perfect. Nobody is. Learn from your experiences and move on.

6. Let go of the past. Stop holding on to what ifs and what could've been. You'll be happier for it.

7. Focus on the present and the future. Be aware of who you are and where you are, and what you want to become.

8. Look at the positive angle. When something doesn't go your way, think of it as an opportunity to get something better instead.

9. Stop thinking too big. Focus on important things like personal relationships and what makes you happy.

10. Be satisfied with what you have. Ambition is good in small doses, but don't let it rule your life. Be grateful for what you have right now.

11. Be patient. Don't think too far ahead. Sometimes, you need to wait for things to unfold first before you take action.

12. Make affirmations when you're upset. These helps you divert negative feelings into positive thoughts.

13. Believe in yourself. If you don't, no one else will.

14. Learn to laugh. Things will begin to lighten up when you laugh.

15. Foster positive relationships. The people around you will always influence your thoughts. Veer away from toxic people.

16. Think of obstacles as challenges. Don't let them overwhelm you; instead, find ways to overcome any and all adversity.

17. Remember that changes are normal and learn to adjust.

18. Be objective. Don't make excuses. Commit yourself to making necessary changes.

19. Think about what you have, not what you don't have. That will make you feel more thankful about who you are.

20. Stay grounded. It's okay to dream, but never forget reality. It helps when you have to deal with disappointments.

30 Ways You Can Sooth Yourself with Distractions

Finally, when the urge to fall back into your old eating habits becomes unbearable, you need distractions to get you going. Here are 30 great suggestions of what you could do when the old craving for a binge returns.

1. Pamper yourself. It doesn't have to be an expensive spa. A relaxing warm bath will work as well to calm your nerves.

2. Aromatherapy. Inhaling certain scents can relax you, such as lavender and rose.

3. Have a cup of tea. The warmth can relieve your tension, and certain herbs like chamomile are known to have soothing properties.

4. Have an apple. Apple is said to calm the nerves.

5. Yoga. You can meditate while you do it.

6. Exercise. Sweat off the tension and stay healthy with a regular routine.

7. Sleep. It rejuvenates you and clears your mind from negative thoughts.

8. Have a mint. Peppermint suppresses your appetite and makes your cravings more manageable.

9. Have a piece of chocolate. A small piece of dark chocolate can be your reward for a stressful day at work, but stop at one piece, and nothing more.

10. Drink some coffee. Coffee is said to have effects on your appetite.

11. Treat yourself to a massage. It relieves muscle tension and lessens your agitation.

12. Go shopping. If you have the money, why not look for the perfect clothes, or how about some shoes? If you don't have money, go window shopping instead.

13. Brain workout. Instead of thinking about food, try out some puzzles instead to divert your attention.

14. Get a hobby. Knitting, scrapbooking or anything to do with your hands will help you drive food away from your mind.

15. Clean your room. It's a great exercise, and sorting out the clutter will definitely take the edge out of your craving.

16. Listen to music. Music can calm your nerves and help you relax.

17. Watch a good movie. It can distract you — as long as you don't snack out while watching.

18. Give your pet some love. Pets are proven stress relievers, and recommended for people with heart ailments and chronic depression.

19. Hang out with a friend. Usually, help is just a call away.

20. Keep a diary or blog. It's great if you want to vent off some spleen without someone suffering at the receiving end.

21. Hug someone. We all need at least six hugs a day to function properly.

22. Help others. Whether it's a soup kitchen or teaching out of school kids, helping out makes you feel good and grateful for what you have.

23. Surround yourself with people. When you don't want to be alone with your thoughts and depression sets in, fight it by having company to distract you.

24. Do some gardening. Plants have therapeutic effects on your disposition.

25. Surf the net. You can find a lot of interesting pieces about all topics you can think of — enough to distract you from grabbing that next cookie.

26. Find creative release. Draw, write, or paint, or anything that channels your energy positively.

27. Play video games. It can help relieve some of your stress and tension.

28. Sing or dance your heart out. Let all those negative emotions out the right way.

29. Go for a walk in a park. It can help clear your head and find something to distract you from food. You can even bring your dog for exercise.

30. Look for support. You could join online forums that help people with eating disorders.

Printed in Great Britain
by Amazon